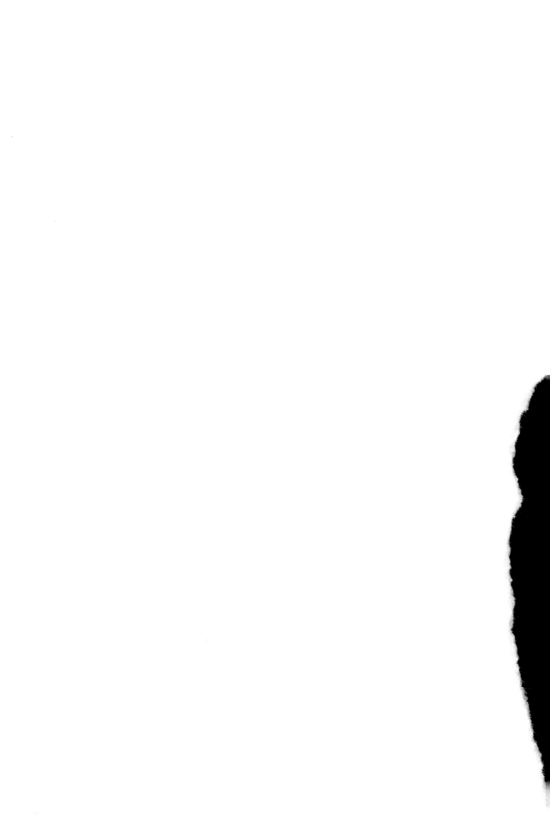

Sommario

5

Introduction

The Mediterranean cuisine has ancient origins, being the cradle of civilization 'has hosted ancient peoples of all kinds and genres, and here in this book I wanted to enclose the best Mediterranean recipes, the recipes more' good and famous, those that were probably invented by ancient peoples who lived there and now are here at your disposal.

But let's not get lost in chitchat and start preparing these delights right away.

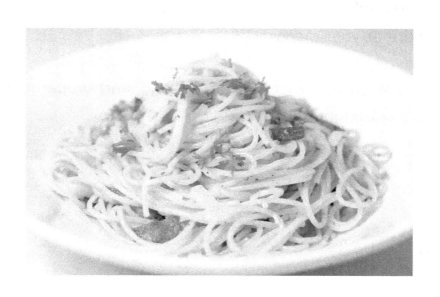

Lunch Recipes

Greek Lemon Chicken Soup

Servings: 8

Cooking Time: 20 Minutes

Ingredients:

- 10 cups chicken broth

- 3 tbsp olive oil

- 8 cloves garlic, minced

- 1 sweet onion

- 1 large lemon, zested

- 2 boneless skinless chicken breasts

- 1 cup Israeli couscous (pearl)

- 1/2 tsp crushed red pepper

- 2 oz crumbled feta

- 1/3 cup chopped chive

- Salt, to taste

- Pepper, to taste

Directions:

1. In a large 6-8-quart sauce pot over medium-low heat, add the olive oil

2. Once heated, sauté the onion and minced the garlic for 3-4 minutes to soften

3. Then add in the chicken broth, raw chicken breasts, lemon zest, and crushed red pepper to the pot Raise the heat to high, cover, and bring to a boil

4. Once boiling, reduce the heat to medium, then simmer for 5 minutes

5. Stir in the couscous, 1 tsp salt, and black pepper to taste

6. Simmer another 5 minute, then turn the heat off

7. Using tongs, remove the two chicken breasts from the pot and transfer to a plate

8. Use a fork and the tongs to shred the chicken, then return to the pot

9. Stir in the crumbled feta cheese and chopped chive

10. Season to taste with salt and pepper as needed

11. Allow the soup to cool completely

12. Distribute among the containers, store for 2-3 days

13. To Serve: Reheat in the microwave for 1-2 minutes or until heated through, or reheat on the stove

Nutrition Info:Per Serving: Calories:2Carbs: 23g;Total Fat: g;Protein: 11g

Mediterranean Steamed Salmon With Fresh Herbs And Lemon

Servings: 4

Cooking Time: 15 Minutes

Ingredients:

- 1 yellow onion, halved and sliced

- 4 green onions spring onions, trimmed and sliced lengthwise, divided

- 1 lb skin-on salmon fillet (such as wild Alaskan), cut into 4 portions

- 1/2 tsp Aleppo pepper

- 4 to 5 garlic cloves, chopped

- Extra virgin olive oil

- A large handful fresh parsley

- 1 lemon, thinly sliced

- 1 tsp ground coriander

- 1 tsp ground cumin

- 1/2 cup white wine (or you can use water or low-sodium broth, if you prefer)

- Kosher salt, to taste

- Black pepper, to taste

Directions:

1. Prepare a large piece of wax paper or parchment paper (about 2 feet long) and place it right in the center of a -inch deep pan or braiser

2. Place the sliced yellow onions and a sprinkle a little bit of green onions the onions on the bottom of the braiser

3. Arrange the salmon, skin-side down, on top, season with kosher salt and black pepper

4. In a small bowl, mix together the coriander, cumin, and Aleppo pepper, coat top of salmon with the spice mixture, and drizzle with a little bit of extra virgin olive oil

5. Then add garlic, parsley and the remaining green onions on top of the salmon (make sure that everything is arrange evenly over the salmon portions.)

6. Arrange the lemon slices on top of the salmon

7. Add another drizzle of extra virgin olive oil, then add the white wine

8. Fold the parchment paper over to cover salmon, secure the edges and cover the braiser with the lid

9. Place the braising pan over medium-high heat, cook for 5 minutes

10. Lower the heat to medium, cook for another 8 minutes, covered still

11. Remove from heat and allow to rest undisturbed for about 5 minutes.

12. Remove the lid and allow the salmon to cool completely

13. Distribute among the containers, store for 2-3 days

14. To Serve: Reheat in the microwave for 1-2 minutes or until heated through.

15. Recipe Notes: The pan or braiser you use needs to have a lid to allow the steamed salmon.

Nutrition Info:Per Serving: Calories:321;Carbs: g;Total Fat: 18g;Protein: 28g

Beef Sausage Pancakes

Servings: 2

Cooking Time: 30 Minutes

Ingredients:

- 4 gluten-free Italian beef sausages, sliced

- 1 tablespoon olive oil

- 1/3 large red bell peppers, seeded and sliced thinly

- 1/3 cup spinach

- ¾ teaspoon garlic powder

- 1/3 large green bell peppers, seeded and sliced thinly

- ¾ cup heavy whipped cream

- Salt and black pepper, to taste

Directions:

1. Mix together all the ingredients in a bowl except whipped cream and keep aside.

2. Put butter and half of the mixture in a skillet and cook for about 6 minutes on both sides.

3. Repeat with the remaining mixture and dish out.

4. Beat whipped cream in another bowl until smooth.

5. Serve the beef sausage pancakes with whipped cream.

6. For meal prepping, it is compulsory to gently slice the sausages before mixing with other ingredients.

Nutrition Info: Calories: 415 ;Carbohydrates: ;Protein: 29.5g;Fat: 31.6g ;Sugar: 4.3g;Sodium: 1040mg

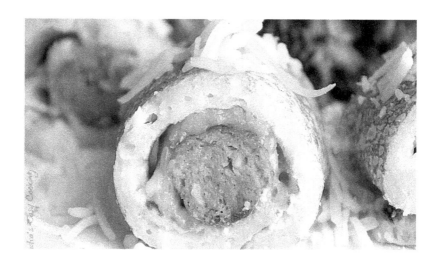

Grilled Salmon Tzatziki Bowl

Servings: 2

Cooking Time: 15 Minutes

Ingredients:

- 8–10 ounces salmon, serves 2

- Olive oil for brushing

- Salt and pepper

- 1 lemon- sliced in half

- Tzatziki:

- ½ cup plain yogurt

- ½ cup sour cream

- 1 garlic clove- finely minced

- 1 tbsp lemon juice, more to taste

- 1 tbsp olive oil

- ½ tsp kosher salt

- ¼ tsp white pepper or black

- ⅛ cup fresh chopped dill (or mint, cilantro or Italian parsley – or a mix)

- 1 ½ cups finely sliced or diced cucumber

- Optional Bowl Additions:

- Cooked Quinoa or rice

- Arugula or other greens

- Grilled veggies like eggplant, peppers, tomatoes, or zucchini

- Fresh veggies of your choice - radishes, cucumber, tomatoes, sprouts

- Garnish with olive oil, lemon, and fresh herbs

Directions:

1. Preheat heat grill to medium high

2. Cook 1 cup quinoa or rice on the stove, according to directions, allow to cool

3. Brush the salmon with olive oil, season with salt and pepper, set aside

4. Create the Tzatziki, by adding plain yogurt, sour cream, garlic clove, lemon juice, olive oil, kosher salt, and white pepper in a bowl, taste and add more lemon juice if desired, store in fridge

5. Place the salmon on the grill, along with the veggies of you choose to grill, brushing all with olive oil, salt and pepper

6. Grill the salmon on both sides for 3-4 minutes, or until cooked through

7. Then grill the lemon, open side down, until good grill marks appear

8. Once the veggies and salmon are done, allow them to cool

9. Distribute among the containers - Divide quinoa among the containers, arrange the grilled vegetables and salmon over top.

10. To Serve: Reheat in the microwave for 1 minute or until heated through. Top with the greens and the fresh veggies, then drizzle a little olive oil on top and season with salt, squeeze the grilled lemon over the whole bowl, spoon the tzatziki over top the salmon, sprinkle with the fresh dill or other herbs. Enjoy with a glass of wine.

Nutrition Info:Per Serving: Calories:458;Carbs: 29g;Total Fat: 24g;Protein: 30g

Smoky Chickpea, Chard, And Butternut Squash Soup

Servings: 8

Cooking Time: 35 Minutes

Ingredients:

- 2 slices bacon (about 1 ounce), chopped

- 1 cup chopped onion

- 1 teaspoon chopped garlic

- 1 teaspoon smoked paprika

- ½ teaspoon kosher salt

- 2 teaspoons fresh thyme leaves, roughly chopped

- 1½ pounds butternut squash, peeled, seeded, and cut into 1-inch cubes

- 1 large bunch chard, stems and leaves chopped

- 2 (15.5-oz) cans low-sodium chickpeas, drained and rinsed

- 32 ounces low-sodium chicken broth

- 1 tablespoon freshly squeezed lemon juice

- 8 teaspoons grated Parmesan or Pecorino Romano cheese for garnish

Directions:

1. Place a soup pot, at least 4½ quarts in size, on the stove over medium heat. Add the chopped bacon and cook until the fat has rendered and the bacon is crisp. Remove the bacon pieces to a plate.

2. Add the chopped onion and garlic to the same pot. Sauté in the bacon fat until the onion is soft, about 5 minutes. Add the paprika, salt, and thyme. Stir to coat the onion well. Add the squash, chard, chickpeas, and broth to the pot.

3. Turn the heat to high, bring the soup to a boil, then turn the heat down to low and simmer until the squash is tender, about 20 minutes.

4. Add the lemon juice. If necessary, add another pinch of salt to taste.

5. Place 2 cups of cooled soup in each of 4 containers and top each serving with 2 teaspoons of cheese. Store the remaining 4 Servings: in the freezer to eat later.

6. STORAGE: Store covered containers in the refrigerator for up to 5 days. If frozen, soup will last 4 months.

Nutrition Info:Per Serving: Total calories: 194; Total fat: 2g; Saturated fat: 1g; Sodium: 530mg; Carbohydrates: 34g; Fiber: 11g; Protein: 12g

Herbed Tuna Salad Wraps

Servings: 4

Cooking Time: 15 Minutes

Ingredients:

- 1 (11-ounce) pouch tuna in water

- 1 cup parsley leaves, chopped

- ¼ cup mint leaves, chopped

- ¼ cup minced shallot

- 1½ teaspoons sumac

- 1 teaspoon Dijon mustard

- 1 tablespoon olive oil

- 1 tablespoon freshly squeezed lemon juice

- ¼ cup unsalted sunflower seeds

- 16 large or medium romaine or bibb lettuce leaves

- 1 red bell pepper, cut into thin sticks (3 to 4 inches long)

- 3 Persian cucumbers, cut into thin sticks (3 to 4 inches long)

Directions:

1. In a large bowl, mix together the tuna, parsley, mint, shallot, sumac, mustard, oil, lemon juice, and sunflower seeds.

2. Place ¾ cup of tuna salad in each of 4 containers. Place 4 lettuce leaves, one quarter of the peppers, and one quarter of the cucumbers in each of 4 separate containers so that they don't get soggy from the tuna salad.

3. STORAGE: Store covered containers in the refrigerator for up to 4 days.

4. TIP Tuna in pouches is preferable to cans, because pouches don't need to be drained and the tuna isn't soggy. You can substitute canned salmon, canned sardines, or even shredded rotisserie chicken for the tuna in this salad.

Nutrition Info:Per Serving: Total calories: 223; Total fat: 9g; Saturated fat: 1g; Sodium: 422mg; Carbohydrates: 12g; Fiber: 4g; Protein: 24g

Mediterranean Potato Salad

Servings: 6

Cooking Time: 30 Minutes

Ingredients:

- 3 tablespoons extra virgin olive oil

- ½ cup of sliced olives

- 1 tablespoon olive juice

- 3 tablespoons lemon juice, freshly squeezed is best

- 2 tablespoons of mint, fresh and torn

- ¼ teaspoon sea salt

- 2 stalks of sliced celery

- 2 pounds baby potatoes

- 2 tablespoons of chopped oregano, fresh is best

Directions:

1. Cut the potatoes into inch cubes.

2. Toss the potatoes into a medium saucepan and cover them with water.

3. Place the saucepan on the stove over high heat.

4. Once the potatoes start to boil, bring the heat down to medium-low.

5. Let the potatoes simmer for 13 to 1minutes. When you poke the potatoes with a fork and they feel tender, they are done.

6. As the potatoes are simmering, grab a small bowl and mix the oil, olive juice, lemon juice, and salt. Whisk the ingredients together well.

7. Once the potatoes are done, drain them and pour the potatoes into a bowl.

8. Take the juice mixture and pour 3 tablespoons over the potatoes right away.

9. Combine the potatoes with the celery and olives.

10. Prior to serving, sprinkle the potatoes with the mint, oregano, and rest of the dressing.

Nutrition Info: calories: 175, fats: 7 grams, carbohydrates: 27 grams, protein: 3 grams.

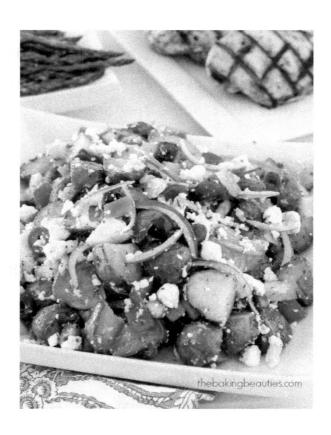

thebakingbeauties.com

Mediterranean Zucchini Noodles

Servings: 2

Cooking Time: 10 Minutes

Ingredients:

- 2 large zucchini or 1 package of store-bought zucchini noodles

- 1 tsp olive oil

- 4 cloves garlic diced

- 10 oz cherry tomatoes cut in half

- 2-4 oz plain hummus

- 1 tsp oregano

- 1/2 tsp red wine vinegar plus more to taste

- 1/2 cup jarred artichoke hearts, drained and chopped

- 1/4 cup sun-dried tomatoes, drained and chopped

- Salt, to taste

- Pepper to taste

- Parmesan and fresh basil for topping

Directions:

1. Prepare the zucchini by cutting of the ends off zucchini and spiralize, set aside

2. In a pan over medium heat, add in olive oil

3. Then add in the garlic and cherry tomatoes to the pan, sauté until tomatoes begin to burst, about to 4 minutes

4. Add in the zucchini noodles, sun-dried tomatoes, hummus, oregano, artichoke hearts and red wine vinegar to the pan, sauté for 1-2 minutes, or until zucchini is tender-crisp and heated through

5. Season to taste with salt and pepper as needed

6. Allow the zoodle to cool

7. Distribute among the containers, store in the fridge for 2-3 days

8. To Serve: Reheat in the microwave for 30 seconds or until heated through, serve immediately with parmesan and fresh basil. Enjoy

Nutrition Info:Per Serving: Calories:241;Carbs: 8g;Total Fat: 37g;Protein: 10g

Lobster Salad

Servings: 2

Cooking Time: 15 Minutes

Ingredients:

- ¼ yellow onion, chopped

- ¼ yellow bell pepper, seeded and chopped

- ¾ pound cooked lobster meat, shredded

- 1 celery stalk, chopped

- Black pepper, to taste

- ¼ cup avocado mayonnaise

Directions:

1. Mix together all the ingredients in a bowl and stir until well combined.

2. Refrigerate for about 3 hours and serve chilled.

3. Put the salad into a container for meal prepping and refrigerate for about 2 days.

Nutrition Info: Calories: 336 ;Carbohydrates: 2g;Protein: 27.2g;Fat: 25.2g ;Sugar: 1.2g;Sodium: 926mg

Mediterranean-style Pesto Chicken

Servings: 4

Cooking Time: 40 Minutes

Ingredients:

- 1 pound chicken breasts (2 large breasts), butterflied and cut in half to make 4 pieces

- 1 (6-ounce) jar prepared pesto

- 1 teaspoon olive oil

- 12 ounces baby spinach leaves

- Chunky Roasted Cherry Tomato and Basil Sauce

Directions:

1. Place the chicken and pesto in a gallon-size resealable bag. Marinate for at least hour.

2. Preheat the oven to 350°F and rub a 13-by-9-inch glass or ceramic baking dish with the oil, or spray with cooking spray.

3. Place the spinach in the pan, then place the chicken on top of the spinach. Pour the pesto from the bag into the dish. Cover the pan with aluminum foil and bake for 20 minutes. Remove the foil and bake for another 15 to 20 minutes. Cool.

4. Place 1 piece of chicken, one quarter of the spinach, and ⅓ cup of chunky tomato sauce in each of separate containers.

5. STORAGE: Store covered containers in the refrigerator for up to days.

Nutrition Info:Per Serving: Total calories: 531; Total fat: 43g; Saturated fat: 7g; Sodium: 1,243mg; Carbohydrates: 13g; Fiber: 4g; Protein: 29g

Crispy Baked Chicken

Servings: 2

Cooking Time: 40 Minutes

Ingredients:

- 2 chicken breasts, skinless and boneless

- 2 tablespoons butter

- ¼ teaspoon turmeric powder

- Salt and black pepper, to taste

- ¼ cup sour cream

Directions:

1. Preheat the oven to 360 degrees F and grease a baking dish with butter.

2. Season the chicken with turmeric powder, salt and black pepper in a bowl.

3. Put the chicken on the baking dish and transfer it in the oven.

4. Bake for about 10 minutes and dish out to serve topped with sour cream.

5. Transfer the chicken in a bowl and set aside to cool for meal prepping. Divide it into 2 containers and cover the containers. Refrigerate for up to 2 days and reheat in microwave before serving.

Nutrition Info: Calories: 304 ;Carbohydrates: 1.4g;Protein: 21g;Fat: 21.6g ;Sugar: 0.1g;Sodium: 137mg

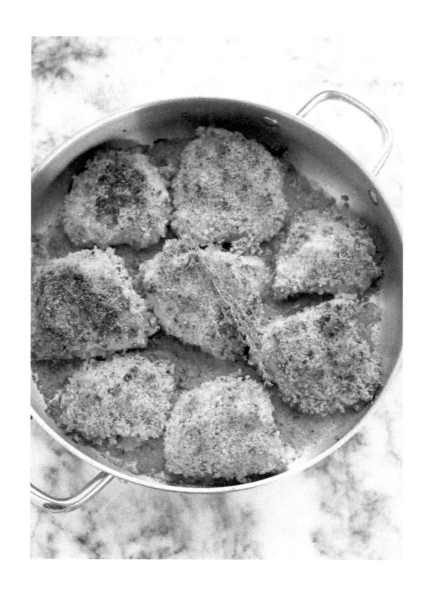

Vegetarian Lasagna Roll-ups

Servings: 14

Cooking Time: 1 Hour 10 Minutes

Ingredients:

- 1 pound lasagna noodles

- 3 thinly sliced zucchini, if your vegetables are smaller make it 4

- ½ cup water

- 3 tablespoons olive oil

- Parmesan cheese and salt to taste

- 24-ounce jar of pasta sauce, you can use any type but the best for the recipes is basil or tomato

- Enough crushed red pepper flakes for your taste buds, this is also optional

- For the cheese filling:

- 6 ounces goat cheese

- 20 ounces of ricotta cheese

- 2 ounces mozzarella cheese

- 1 cup of parsley leaves, chopped

- Dash of salt and pepper

- 3 tablespoons of chopped garlic

- Olive oil

Directions:

1. Set the temperature of your oven to 450 degrees Fahrenheit.

2. Grease a baking sheet or lay a piece of parchment paper on top.

3. Slice the zucchini and place them on the baking sheet.

4. Brush each side of the vegetable with oil and then sprinkle with salt.

5. Place the baking sheet into the oven and set a timer for 10 minutes.

6. While the zucchini is baking, start boiling the lasagna noodles. Drain the noodles when they are done cooking and then let them dry on a piece of parchment paper.

7. Remove the zucchini from the oven and set aside to allow them to cool down a bit.

8. Change the heat of your oven to 350 degrees Fahrenheit.

9. To make the cheese filling, combine all of the ingredients and drizzle with a little olive oil. Mix well.

10. Pour a spoonful or two on each of the lasagna noodles.

11.   Set a slice of baked zucchini on top of the cheese mixture.

12.   Roll up the noodles.

13.   In a 9 x inch baking pan, pour the water and ¾ cup of the pasta sauce on the bottom. Stir the ingredients gently so they become mixed.

14.   Place the lasagna roll-ups in the upright position on top of the sauce.

15.   Pour the remaining sauce on the noodles.

16.   If you want a little extra cheese, sprinkle some on top of the lasagna roll-ups.

17.   Set your timer for 40 minutes, but remember to check the liquid half-way through cooking to make sure it does not become too dry. If it does, add a little more water. You can try adding some water to the pasta sauce jar and shaking it up a bit as this will give the water a little sauce flavor.

18. When the lasagna is cooked, remove it and garnish with basil leaves. Allow it to cool for a couple of minutes and admire your Mediterranean cooking skills before serving.

Nutrition Info: calories: 282, fats: 11 grams, carbohydrates: 29 grams, protein: 14.3 grams.

Milano Chicken

Servings: 6

Cooking Time: 30 Minutes

Ingredients:

- 4 skinless and boneless chicken breast halves

- 1 tablespoon vegetable oil

- 2 garlic cloves, crushed

- 1 teaspoon Italian style seasoning

- 1 teaspoon crushed red pepper flakes

- salt

- pepper

- 1 28-ounce can stewed drained tomatoes

- 1 9-ounce package frozen green beans

Directions:

1. Heat oil in a large skillet over medium-high heat.

2. Add chicken to the skillet and season with garlic, red pepper, Italian seasoning, salt, and pepper.

3. Saute for about 5 minutes.

4. Add tomatoes and cook for 5 minutes more.

5. Add green beans and give the whole mixture a gentle stir.

6. Reduce heat, cover, and simmer for about 15-20 minutes.

7. Enjoy!

Nutrition Info:Per Serving: Calories: 244, Total Fat: 4.9 g, Saturated Fat: 0.5 g, Cholesterol: mg, Sodium: 399 mg, Total Carbohydrate: 14.1 g, Dietary Fiber: 4.6 g, Total Sugars: 6.4 g, Protein: 38.2 g,

Vitamin D: 0 mcg, Calcium: 48 mg, Iron: 3 mg, Potassium: 662 mg

Tuna Celery Salad

Servings: 4

Cooking Time: 30 Minutes

Ingredients:

- 3 5-ounce cans Genova tuna dipped in olive oil

- 2½ celery stalks, chopped

- ½ English cucumber, chopped

- 4-5 small radishes, stems removed, chopped

- 3 green onions, chopped (white and green)

- ½ medium red onion, finely chopped

- ½ cup pitted Kalamata olives, halved

- 1 bunch parsley, stems removed, finely chopped

- 10-15 sprigs fresh mint leaves, stems removed, finely chopped

- 6 slices heirloom tomatoes

- pita chips or pita bread

- 2½ teaspoons high-quality Dijon mustard

- zest of 1 lime

- lime juice, 1½ limes

- 1/3 cup olive oil

- ½ teaspoon sumac

- salt

- pepper

- ½ teaspoon crushed red pepper flakes

Directions:

1. Prepare the vinaigrette by combining and whisking all zesty Dijon mustard vinaigrette Ingredients: in a small bowl.

2. For the tuna salad, add all base recipe Ingredients: to a large bowl, and mix well with a spoon.

3. Dress the tuna salad with the prepared vinaigrette, and mix again until the tuna salad is coated correctly.

4. Cover, refrigerate and allow to chill for 30 minutes.

5. Once chilled, give the salad a toss and serve with a side of pita chips or pita bread and some sliced up heirloom tomatoes.

6. Enjoy!

Nutrition Info:Per Serving: Calories: 455, Total Fat: 33.8 g, Saturated Fat: 5.9 g, Cholesterol: 3mg,

Sodium: 832 mg, Total Carbohydrate: 20.1 g, Dietary Fiber: 6.3 g, Total Sugars: 4 g, Protein: 24.3 g, Vitamin D: 0 mcg, Calcium: 155 mg, Iron: 7 mg, Potassium: 604 mg

Chicken With Herbed Butter

Servings: 2

Cooking Time: 35 Minutes

Ingredients:

- 1/3 cup baby spinach

- 1 tablespoon lemon juice

- ¾ pound chicken breasts

- 1/3 cup butter

- ¼ cup parsley, chopped

- Salt and black pepper, to taste

- 1/3 teaspoon ginger powder

- 1 garlic clove, minced

Directions:

1. Preheat the oven to 450 degrees F and grease a baking dish.

2. Mix together parsley, ginger powder, lemon juice, butter, garlic, salt and black pepper in a bowl.

3. Add chicken breasts in the mixture and marinate well for about minutes.

4. Arrange the marinated chicken in the baking dish and transfer in the oven.

5. Bake for about 2minutes and dish out to serve immediately.

6. Place chicken in 2 containers and refrigerate for about 3 days for meal prepping. Reheat in microwave before serving.

Nutrition Info: Calories: 568 ;Carbohydrates: 1.6g;Protein: 44.6g;Fat: 42.1g;Sugar: 0.3g;Sodium: 384mg

Italian Tuna Sandwiches

Servings: 4

Cooking Time: 10 Minutes

Ingredients:

- 3 tablespoons lemon juice, freshly squeezed

- ½ teaspoon of minced garlic

- 5 ounces tuna, drained

- ½ cup of sliced olives

- 8 slices whole-grain bread

- 2 tablespoons extra virgin olive oil

- ½ teaspoon black pepper

- 1 celery stalk, chopped

Directions:

1. Add the oil, pepper, lemon juice, and garlic to a bowl. Whisk the ingredients well.

2. Combine the olives, chopped celery, and tuna.

3. Use a fork to break apart the tuna into chunks.

4. Stir all of the ingredients until they are well combined.

5. Set four slices of bread on serving plates or a platter.

6. Divide the tuna salad equally among the four slices of bread.

7. Top the tuna salad with the remaining bread to make a sandwich.

8. You'll get the best taste when you let the tuna sandwich sit for about 5 or more minutes before you serve. The salad will start to soak into the bread, and it makes for one tasty meal!

Nutrition Info: calories: 347, fats: 17 grams, carbohydrates: 27 grams, protein: 25 grams.

Mediterranean Baked Sole Fillet

Servings: 6

Cooking Time: 15 Minutes

Ingredients:

- 1 lime or lemon, juice of

- 1/2 cup extra virgin olive oil

- 3 tbsp unsalted melted vegan butter

- 2 shallots, thinly sliced

- 3 garlic cloves, thinly-sliced

- 2 tbsp capers

- 1.5 lb Sole fillet, about 10–12 thin fillets

- 4–6 green onions, top trimmed, halved lengthwise

- 1 lime or lemon, sliced (optional)

- 3/4 cup roughly chopped fresh dill for garnish

- 1 tsp seasoned salt, or to your taste

- 3/4 tsp ground black pepper

- 1 tsp ground cumin

- 1 tsp garlic powder

Directions:

1. Preheat over to 375-degree F

2. In a small bowl, whisk together olive oil, lime juice, and melted butter with a sprinkle of seasoned salt, stir in the garlic, shallots, and capers.

3. In a separate small bowl, mix together the pepper, cumin, seasoned salt, and garlic powder, season the fish fillets each on both sides

4. On a large baking pan or dish, arrange the fish fillets and cover with the buttery lime

5. Arrange the green onion halves and lime slices on top

6. Bake in 375 degrees F for 10-15 minutes, do not overcook

7. Remove the fish fillets from the oven

8. Allow the dish to cool completely

9. Distribute among the containers, store for 2-3 days

10. To Serve: Reheat in the microwave for 1-2 minutes or until heated through. Garnish with the chopped fresh dill. Serve with your favorite and a fresh salad

11. Recipe Notes: If you can't get your hands on a sole fillet, cook this recipe with a different white fish. Just remember to change the baking time since it will be different.

Nutrition Info:Per Serving: Calories:350;Carbs:7 g;Total Fat: 26g;Protein: 23g

Baked Chicken Breast

Servings: 2

Cooking Time: 50 Minutes

Ingredients:

- 2 skinless and boneless chicken breasts (about 8 ounces each)

- salt

- ground black pepper

- ¼ cup olive oil

- ¼ cup freshly squeezed lemon juice

- 1 garlic clove, minced

- ½ teaspoon dried oregano

- ¼ teaspoon dried thyme

Directions:

1. Preheat oven to a temperature of 400 degrees F.

2. Season the chicken breasts carefully with salt and pepper on all sides.

3. Place the chicken in a bowl.

4. Take another bowl and add olive oil, lemon juice, oregano, garlic, and thyme. Mix well to make the marinade.

5. Pour the marinade on top of chicken breasts and allow to marinate for 10 minutes.

6. Set an oven rack about inches above the heat source.

7. Place the chicken breasts into a baking pan and pour extra marinade on top.

8. Bake for about 35-45 minutes until the center is no longer pink and the juices run clear.

9. Move the baking dish to top rack and broil for about 5 minutes.

10.   Cool, spread over containers with some side dish and enjoy!

Nutrition Info:Per Serving: Calories: 467, Total Fat: 28.5 g, Saturated Fat: 3.9 g, Cholesterol: 130 mg, Sodium: 158 mg, Total Carbohydrate: 1.5 g, Dietary Fiber: 0.4 g, Total Sugars: 0.7 g, Protein: 52.4 g, Vitamin D: 0 mcg, Calcium: 14 mg, Iron: 2 mg, Potassium: 52 mg

Grilled Lemon Fish

Servings: 4

Cooking Time: 15 Minutes

Ingredients:

- ¼ teaspoon sea salt

- 3 to 4 lemons

- ¼ teaspoon ground black pepper

- 4 ounces any fish fillets, such as salmon or cod

- 1 tablespoon olive oil

Directions:

1. Ensure that the fish fillets are dry. If you know or feel they are a bit damp, take a paper towel and pat them dry.

2. Leave the fish fillets on the counter for 10 minutes so they can stand at room temperature.

3. Turn on your grill to medium-high heat or set the temperature to 400 degrees Fahrenheit.

4. Using nonstick cooking spray, coat the grill so the fish won't stick.

5. Take one lemon and cut it in half. Set one of the halves aside and cut the remaining half into ¼-inch thick slices.

6. Now, take the other half of the lemon and squeeze at least 1 tablespoon of juice out into a small bowl.

7. Add oil into the small bowl and whisk the ingredients together.

8. Brush the fish with the lemon and oil mixture. Make sure you get both sides of the fish.

9. Arrange the lemon slices on the grill in the shape of the fish, it might take about 3 to 4 slices for one fish.

10. Place the fish on top of the lemon slices and grill the ingredients together. If you don't have a lid for your grill, cover it with a different lid that will fit or use aluminum foil.

11. When the fish is about half-way done, turn it over so the other side is laying on top of the lemon slices.

12. You will know the fish is done when it starts to look flaky and separates easily, which you can check by gently pressing a fork onto the fish.

Nutrition Info: calories: 147, fats: 5 grams, carbohydrates: 4 grams, protein: 22 grams.

Italian Baked Beans

Servings: 6

Cooking Time: 15 To 20 Minutes.

Ingredients:

- ½ cup chopped onion

- ¼ cup red wine vinegar

- ¼ tablespoon ground cinnamon

- 15 ounces or 2 cans of great northern beans, do not drain

- 2 teaspoons extra virgin olive oil

- 12 ounces tomato paste, low sodium

- ½ cup water

Directions:

1. Turn a burner to medium heat and add oil to a saucepan.

2. Add the onion and cook for 4 to 5 minutes. Stir well.

3. Combine the vinegar, tomato paste, cinnamon, and water. Mix until all the ingredients are well combined.

4. Switch the heat to a low setting.

5. Using a colander, drain one can of beans and pour into the pan.

6. Open the second can of beans and pour all of it, including the liquid, into the saucepan and stir.

7. Continue to cook the beans for 10 minutes while stirring frequently.

8. Serve and enjoy!

Nutrition Info: calories: 236, fats: 3 grams, carbohydrates: 42 grams, protein: 10 grams.

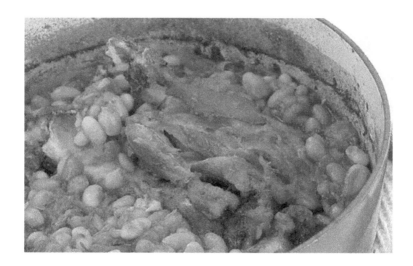

Tomato Tilapia

Servings: 4

Cooking Time: 15 Minutes

Ingredients:

- 3 tablespoons sun-dried tomatoes packed in oil, drained (juice/oil reserved) and chopped

- 1 tablespoon capers, drained

- 2 pieces tilapia

- 1 tablespoon oil from sun-dried tomatoes

- 1 tablespoon lemon juice

- 2 tablespoons Kalamata olives, pitted and chopped

Directions:

1. Preheat oven to 375 degrees F.

2. Add sun-dried tomatoes, capers, and olives to a bowl; stir well and set aside.

3. Place the tilapia fillets side by side on a baking sheet.

4. Drizzle with oil and lemon juice.

5. Bake for about 10-1minutes.

6. Check the fish after 10 minutes to see if they are flakey.

7. Once done, top the fish with tomato mixture.

Nutrition Info:Per Serving: Calories: , Total Fat: 4.4 g, Saturated Fat: 0.8 g, Cholesterol: 28 mg, Sodium: 122 mg, Total Carbohydrate: 0.8 g, Dietary Fiber: 0.3 g, Total Sugars: 0.3 g, Protein: 10.7 g, Vitamin D: 0 mcg, Calcium: 16 mg, Iron: 1 mg, Potassium: 26 mg

Chicken Lentil Soup

Servings: 4

Cooking Time: 45 Minutes

Ingredients:

- 1 pound dried lentils

- 12 ounces boneless chicken thigh meat

- 7 cups water

- 1 small onion, diced

- 2 scallions, chopped

- ¼ cup chopped cilantro

- 3 cloves garlic

- 1 medium tomato, diced

- 1 teaspoon garlic powder

- 1 teaspoon cumin

- ¼ teaspoon oregano

- ½ teaspoon paprika

- ½ teaspoon kosher salt

Directions:

1. Add all of the listed Ingredients: to your Instant Pot.

2. Set your pot to SOUP mode and cook for 30 minutes.

3. Allow the pressure to release naturally.

4. Take the chicken out and shred.

5. Place the chicken back in the pot and stir.

6. Pour to the jars.

7. Enjoy!

Nutrition Info:Per Serving: Calories: 1144, Total Fat: 52.5 g, Saturated Fat: 15.2 g, Cholesterol: 2 mg, Sodium: 558 mg, Total Carbohydrate: 73.2 g, Dietary Fiber: 35.9 g, Total Sugars: 4.3 g, Protein: 90.3 g, Vitamin D: 0 mcg, Calcium: 148 mg, Iron: 13 mg, Potassium: 1241 mg

Bacon Wrapped Asparagus

Servings: 2

Cooking Time: 30 Minutes

Ingredients:

- 1/3 cup heavy whipping cream

- 2 bacon slices, precooked

- 4 small spears asparagus

- Salt, to taste

- 1 tablespoon butter

Directions:

1. Preheat the oven to 360 degrees F and grease a baking sheet with butter.

2. Meanwhile, mix cream, asparagus and salt in a bowl.

3. Wrap the asparagus in bacon slices and arrange them in the baking dish.

4. Transfer the baking dish in the oven and bake for about 20 minutes.

5. Remove from the oven and serve hot.

6. Place the bacon wrapped asparagus in a dish and set aside to cool for meal prepping. Divide it in 2 containers and cover the lid. Refrigerate for about 2 days and reheat in the microwave before serving.

Nutrition Info: Calories: 204 ;Carbohydrates: 1.4g;Protein: 5.9g;Fat: 19.3g;Sugar: 0.5g;Sodium: 291mg

Cool Mediterranean Fish

Servings: 8

Cooking Time: 30 Minutes

Ingredients:

- 6 ounces halibut fillets

- 1 tablespoon Greek seasoning

- 1 large tomato, chopped

- 1 onion, chopped

- 5 ounces kalamata olives, pitted

- ¼ cup capers

- ¼ cup olive oil

- 1 tablespoon lemon juice

- Salt and pepper as needed

Directions:

1. Pre-heat your oven to 350-degree Fahrenheit

2. Transfer the halibut fillets on a large aluminum foil

3. Season with Greek seasoning

4. Take a bowl and add tomato, onion, olives, olive oil, capers, pepper, lemon juice and salt

5. Mix well and spoon the tomato mix over the halibut

6. Seal the edges and fold to make a packet

7. Place the packet on a baking sheet and bake in your oven for 30-40 minutes

8. Serve once the fish flakes off and enjoy!

9. Meal Prep/Storage Options: Store in airtight containers in your fridge for 1-2 days.

Nutrition Info: Calories: 429;Fat: 26g;
Carbohydrates: ; Protein:36g

Luncheon Fancy Salad

Servings: 2

Cooking Time: 40 Minutes

Ingredients:

- 6-ounce cooked salmon, chopped

- 1 tablespoon fresh dill, chopped

- Salt and black pepper, to taste

- 4 hard-boiled grass-fed eggs, peeled and cubed

- 2 celery stalks, chopped

- ½ yellow onion, chopped

- ¾ cup avocado mayonnaise

Directions:

1. Put all the ingredients in a bowl and mix until well combined.

2. Cover with a plastic wrap and refrigerate for about 3 hours to serve.

3. For meal prepping, put the salad in a container and refrigerate for up to days.

Nutrition Info: Calories: 303 ;Carbohydrates: 1.7g;Protein: 10.3g;Fat: 30g ;Sugar: 1g;Sodium: 31g

Moroccan Spiced Stir-fried Beef With Butternut Squash And Chickpeas

Servings: 4

Cooking Time: 15 Minutes

Ingredients:

- 1 tablespoon olive oil, plus 2 teaspoons

- 1 pound precut butternut squash cut into ½-inch cubes

- 3 ounces scallions, white and green parts chopped (1 cup)

- 1 tablespoon water

- ¼ teaspoon baking soda

- ¾ pound flank steak, sliced across the grain into ⅛-inch thick slices

- ½ teaspoon garlic powder

- ¼ teaspoon ground ginger

- ¼ teaspoon turmeric

- ¼ teaspoon ground cumin

- ¼ teaspoon ground coriander

- ⅛ teaspoon cayenne pepper

- ⅛ teaspoon ground cinnamon

- ½ teaspoon kosher salt, divided

- 1 (14-ounce) can chickpeas, drained and rinsed

- ½ cup dried apricots, quartered

- ½ cup cilantro leaves, chopped

- 2 teaspoons freshly squeezed lemon juice

- 8 teaspoons sliced almonds

Directions:

1. Heat tablespoon of oil in a 12-inch skillet. Once the oil is hot, add the squash and scallions, and cook until the squash is tender, about 10 to 12 minutes.

2. Mix the water and baking soda together in a small prep bowl. Place the beef in a medium bowl, pour the baking-soda water over it, and mix to combine. Let it sit for 5 minutes.

3. In a small bowl, combine the garlic powder, ginger, turmeric, cumin, coriander, cayenne, cinnamon, and ¼ teaspoon of salt, then add the mixture to the beef. Stir to combine.

4. When the squash is tender, turn the heat off and add the remaining ¼ teaspoon of salt and the chickpeas, dried apricots, cilantro, and lemon juice to taste. Stir to combine. Place the contents of the pan in a bowl to cool.

5. Clean out the skillet and heat the remaining 2 teaspoons of oil over high heat. When the oil is hot, add the beef and cook until it is no longer pink, about 2 to 3 minutes.

6. Place 1¼ cups of the squash mixture and one quarter of the beef slices in each of 4 containers. Sprinkle 2 teaspoons of sliced almonds over each container.

7. STORAGE: Store covered containers in the refrigerator for up to 5 days.

Nutrition Info:Per Serving: Total calories: 404; Total fat: 14g; Saturated fat: 1g; Sodium: 355mg; Carbohydrates: 46g; Fiber: 12g; Protein: 27g

North African–inspired Sautéed Shrimp With Leeks And Peppers

Servings: 4

Cooking Time: 20 Minutes

Ingredients:

- 2 tablespoons olive oil, divided

- 1 large leek, white and light green parts, halved lengthwise, sliced ¼-inch thick

- 2 teaspoons chopped garlic

- 1 large red bell pepper, chopped into ¼-inch pieces

- 1 cup chopped fresh parsley leaves (1 small bunch)

- ½ cup chopped fresh cilantro leaves (½ small bunch)

- ¼ teaspoon ground cumin

- ¼ teaspoon ground coriander

- 1 teaspoon smoked paprika

- 1 pound uncooked peeled, deveined large shrimp (20 to 25 per pound), thawed if frozen, blotted with paper towels

- 1 tablespoon freshly squeezed lemon juice

- ⅛ teaspoon kosher salt

Directions:

1. Heat 2 teaspoons of oil in a -inch skillet over medium heat. Once the oil is hot, add the leeks and garlic and sauté for 2 minutes. Add the peppers and cook for 10 minutes, or until the peppers are soft, stirring occasionally.

2. Add the chopped parsley and cilantro and cook for 1 more minute. Remove the mixture from the pan and place in a medium bowl.

3. Mix the cumin, coriander, and paprika in a small prep bowl.

4. Add 2 teaspoons of oil to the same skillet and increase the heat to medium-high. Add the shrimp in a single layer, sprinkle the spice mixture over the shrimp, and cook for about 2 minutes. Flip the shrimp over and cook for 1 more minute. Add the leek and herb mixture, stir, and cook for 1 more minute.

5. Turn off the heat and add the remaining 2 teaspoons of oil and the lemon juice. Taste to see whether you need the salt. Add if necessary.

6. Place ¾ cup of couscous or other grain (if using) and 1 cup of the shrimp mixture in each of 4 containers.

7. STORAGE: Store covered containers in the refrigerator for up to 4 days.

Nutrition Info:Per Serving: Total calories: 1; Total fat: 9g; Saturated fat: 1g; Sodium: 403mg; Carbohydrates: 9g; Fiber: 2g; Protein: 19g

Italian Chicken With Sweet Potato And Broccoli

Servings: 8

Cooking Time: 30 Minutes

Ingredients:

- 2 lbs boneless skinless chicken breasts, cut into small pieces

- 5-6 cups broccoli florets

- 3 tbsp Italian seasoning mix of your choice

- a few tbsp of olive oil

- 3 sweet potatoes, peeled and diced

- Coarse sea salt, to taste

- Freshly cracked pepper, to taste

- Toppings:

- Avocado

- Lemon juice

- Chives

- Olive oil, for serving

Directions:

1. Preheat the oven to 425 degrees F

2. Toss the chicken pieces with the Italian seasoning mix and a drizzle of olive oil, stir to combine then store in the fridge for about 30 minutes

3. Arrange the broccoli florets and sweet potatoes on a sheet pan, drizzle with the olive oil, sprinkle generously with salt

4. Arrange the chicken on a separate sheet pan

5. Bake both in the oven for 12-1minutes

6. Transfer the chicken and broccoli to a plate, toss the sweet potatoes and continue to roast for another 15 minutes, or until ready

7. Allow the chicken, broccoli, and sweet potatoes to cool

8. Distribute among the containers and store for 2-3 days

9. To Serve: Reheat in the microwave for 1 minute or until heated through, top with the topping of choice. Enjoy

10. Recipe Notes: Any kind of vegetables work will with this recipe! So, add favorites like carrots, brussels sprouts and asparagus.

Nutrition Info:Per Serving: Calories:222;Total Fat: 4.9g;Total Carbs: 15.3g;Protein: 28g

Vegetable Soup

Servings: 6

Cooking Time: 20 Minutes

Ingredients:

- 1 15-ounce can low sodium cannellini beans, drained and rinsed

- 1 tablespoon olive oil

- 1 small onion, diced

- 2 carrots, diced

- 2 stalks celery, diced

- 1 small zucchini, diced

- 1 garlic clove, minced

- 1 tablespoon fresh thyme leaves, chopped

- 2 teaspoons fresh sage, chopped

- ½ teaspoon salt

- ¼ teaspoon freshly ground black pepper

- 32 ounces low sodium chicken broth

- 1 14-ounce can no-salt diced tomatoes, undrained

- 2 cups baby spinach leaves, chopped

- 1/3 cup freshly grated parmesan

Directions:

1. Mash half of the beans in a small bowl using the back of a spoon and put it to the side.

2. Add the oil to a large soup pot and place over medium-high heat.

3. Add carrots, onion, celery, garlic, zucchini, thyme, salt, pepper, and sage.

4. Cook well for about 5 minutes until the vegetables are tender.

5. Add broth and tomatoes and bring the mixture to a boil.

6. Add beans (both mashed and whole) and spinach.

7. Cook for 3 minutes until the spinach has wilted.

8. Pour the soup into the jars.

9. Before serving, top with parmesan.

10. Enjoy!

Nutrition Info:Per Serving: Calories: 359, Total Fat: 7.1 g, Saturated Fat: 2.7 g, Cholesterol: 10 mg, Sodium: 854 mg, Total Carbohydrate: 51.1 g, Dietary Fiber: 20 g, Total Sugars: 5.7 g, Protein: 25.8 g, Vitamin D: 0 mcg, Calcium: 277 mg, Iron: 7 mg, Potassium: 1497 mg

Greek Chicken Wraps

Servings: 2

Cooking Time: 15 Minutes

Ingredients:

- Greek Chicken Wrap Filling:

- 2 chicken breasts 14 oz, chopped into 1-inch pieces

- 2 small zucchinis, cut into 1-inch pieces

- 2 bell peppers, cut into 1-inch pieces

- 1 red onion, cut into 1-inch pieces

- 2 tbsp olive oil

- 2 tsp oregano

- 2 tsp basil

- 1/2 tsp garlic powder

- 1/2 tsp onion powder

- 1/2 tsp salt

- 2 lemons, sliced

- To Serve:

- 1/4 cup feta cheese crumbled

- 4 large flour tortillas or wraps

Directions:

1. Pre-heat oven to 425 degrees F

2. In a bowl, toss together the chicken, zucchinis, olive oil, oregano, basil, garlic, bell peppers, onion powder, onion powder and salt

3. Arrange lemon slice on the baking sheet(s), spread the chicken and vegetable out on top (use 2 baking sheets if needed)

4. Bake for 15 minutes, until veggies are soft and the chicken is cooked through

5. Allow to cool completely

6. Distribute the chicken, bell pepper, zucchini and onions among the containers and remove the lemon slices

7. Allow the dish to cool completely

8. Distribute among the containers, store for 3 days

9. To Serve: Reheat in the microwave for 1-2 minutes or until heated through. Wrap in a tortila and sprinkle with feta cheese. Enjoy!

Nutrition Info:Per Serving: (1 wrap): Calories:356;Total Fat: 14g;Total Carbs: 26g;Protein: 29g

Garbanzo Bean Soup

Servings: 4

Cooking Time: 20 Minutes

Ingredients:

- 14 ounces diced tomatoes

- 1 teaspoon olive oil

- 1 15-ounce can garbanzo beans

- salt

- pepper

- 2 sprigs fresh rosemary

- 1 cup acini di pepe pasta

Directions:

1. Take a large saucepan and add tomatoes and ounces of the beans.

2. Bring the mixture to a boil over medium-high heat.

3. Puree the remaining beans in a blender/food processor.

4. Stir the pureed mixture into the pan.

5. Add the sprigs of rosemary to the pan.

6. Add acini de Pepe pasta and simmer until the pasta is soft, making sure to stir it from time to time.

7. Remove the rosemary.

8. Season with pepper and salt.

9. Enjoy!

Nutrition Info:Per Serving: Calories: 473, Total Fat: 8.6 g, Saturated Fat: 1.1 g, Cholesterol: 18 mg, Sodium: 66 mg, Total Carbohydrate: 78.8 g, Dietary Fiber: 19.9 g, Total Sugars: 14 g, Protein: 23.7 g,

Vitamin D: 0 mcg, Calcium: 131 mg, Iron: 8 mg, Potassium: 1186 mg

Spinach And Beans Mediterranean Style Salad

Servings: 4

Cooking Time: 30 Minutes

Ingredients:

- 15 ounces drained and rinsed cannellini beans

- 14 ounces drained, rinsed, and quartered artichoke hearts

- 6 ounces or 8 cups baby spinach

- 14 ½ ounces undrained diced tomatoes, no salt is best

- 1 tablespoon olive oil and any additional if you prefer

- ¼ teaspoon salt

- 2 minced garlic cloves

- 1 chopped onion, small in size

- ¼ teaspoon pepper

- ⅛ teaspoon crushed red pepper flakes

- 2 tablespoons Worcestershire sauce

Directions:

1. Place a saucepan on your stovetop and turn the temperature to medium-high.

2. Let the pan warm up for a minute before you pour in the tablespoon of oil. Continue to let the oil heat up for another minute or two.

3. Toss in your chopped onion and stir so all the pieces are bathed in oil. Saute the onions for minutes.

4. Add the garlic to the saucepan. Stir and saute the ingredients for another minute.

5. Combine the salt, red pepper flakes, pepper, and Worcestershire sauce. Mix well and then

add the tomatoes to the pan. Stir the mixture constantly for about minutes.

6. Add the artichoke hearts, spinach, and beans. Saute and stir occasionally to get the taste throughout the dish. Once the spinach starts to wilt, take the salad off of the heat.

7. Serve and enjoy immediately to get the best taste.

Nutrition Info: calories: 1, fats: 4 grams, carbohydrates: 30 grams, protein: 8 grams.

Salmon Skillet Dinner

Servings: 4

Cooking Time: 15 To 20 Minutes

Ingredients:

- 1 teaspoon minced garlic

- 1 ½ cup quartered cherry tomatoes

- 1 tablespoon water

- ¼ teaspoon sea salt

- 1 tablespoon lemon juice, freshly squeezed is best

- 1 tablespoon extra virgin olive oil

- 12 ounces drained and chopped roasted red peppers

- 1 teaspoon paprika

- ¼ teaspoon black pepper

- 1 pound salmon fillets

Directions:

1. Remove the skin from your salmon fillets and cut them into 8 pieces.

2. Turn your stove burner on medium heat and set a skillet on top.

3. Pour the olive oil into the skillet and let it heat up for a couple of minutes.

4. Add the minced garlic and paprika. Saute the ingredients for 1 minute.

5. Combine the roasted peppers, black pepper, tomatoes, water, and salt.

6. Set the heat to medium-high and bring the ingredients to a simmer. This should take 3 to 4 minutes. Remember to stir the ingredients occasionally so the tomatoes don't burn.

7. Add the salmon and take some of the sauce from the skillet to spoon on top of the fish so it is all covered in the mixture.

8. Cover the skillet and set a timer for 10 minutes. When the fish reaches 145 degrees Fahrenheit, it is cooked thoroughly.

9. Turn off the heat and drizzle lemon juice over the fish.

10. Break up the salmon into chunks and gently mix the pieces of fish with the sauce.

11. Serve and enjoy!

Nutrition Info: calories: 289, fats: 13 grams, carbohydrates: 10 grams, protein: 31 grams.

Herb-crusted Halibut

Servings: 4

Cooking Time: 25 Minutes

Ingredients:

- Fresh parsley (.33 cup)

- Fresh dill (.25 cup)

- Fresh chives (.25 cup)

- Lemon zest (1 tsp.)

- Panko breadcrumbs (.75 cup)

- Olive oil (1 tbsp.)

- Freshly cracked black pepper (.25 tsp.)

- Sea salt (1 tsp.)

- Halibut fillets (4 - 6 oz.)

Directions:

1. Chop the fresh dill, chives, and parsley. Prepare a baking tray using a sheet of foil. Set the oven to reach 400° Fahrenheit.

2. Combine the salt, pepper, lemon zest, olive oil, chives, dill, parsley, and the breadcrumbs in a mixing bowl.

3. Rinse the halibut thoroughly. Use paper towels to dry it before baking.

4. Arrange the fish on the baking sheet. Spoon the crumbs over the fish and press it into each of the fillets.

5. Bake it until the top is browned and easily flaked or about 10 to 1minutes.

Nutrition Info: Calories: 273;Protein: 38 grams;Fat: 7 grams

Syrian Spiced Lentil, Barley, And Vegetable Soup

Servings: 5

Cooking Time: 40 Minutes

Ingredients:

- 1 tablespoon olive oil

- 1 small onion, chopped (about 2 cups)

- 2 medium carrots, peeled and chopped (about 1 cup)

- 1 celery stalk, chopped (about ½ cup)

- 1 teaspoon chopped garlic

- 1 teaspoon ground cumin

- 1 teaspoon ground coriander

- 1 teaspoon turmeric

- ⅛ teaspoon ground cinnamon

- 2 tablespoons tomato paste

- ¾ cup green lentils

- ¾ cup pearled barley

- 8 cups water

- ¾ teaspoon kosher salt

- 1 (5-ounce) package baby spinach leaves

- 2 teaspoons red wine vinegar

Directions:

1. Heat the oil in a soup pot on medium-high heat. When the oil is shimmering, add the onion, carrots, celery, and garlic and sauté for 8 minutes. Add the cumin, coriander, turmeric, cinnamon, and tomato paste and cook for 2 more minutes, stirring frequently.

2. Add the lentils, barley, water, and salt to the pot and bring to a boil. Turn the heat to low and

simmer for minutes. Add the spinach and continue to simmer for 5 more minutes.

3. Add the vinegar and adjust the seasoning if needed.

4. Spoon 2 cups of soup into each of 5 containers.

5. STORAGE: Store covered containers in the refrigerator for up to days.

Nutrition Info:Per Serving: Total calories: 273; Total fat: 4g; Saturated fat: 1g; Sodium: 459mg; Carbohydrates: 50g; Fiber: 1; Protein: 12g

Spinach Chicken

Servings: 2

Cooking Time: 20 Minutes

Ingredients:

- 2 garlic cloves, minced

- 2 tablespoons unsalted butter, divided

- ¼ cup parmesan cheese, shredded

- ¾ pound chicken tenders

- ¼ cup heavy cream

- 10 ounce frozen spinach, chopped

- Salt and black pepper, to taste

Directions:

1. Heat tablespoon of butter in a large skillet and add chicken, salt and black pepper.

2. Cook for about 3 minutes on both sides and remove the chicken in a bowl.

3. Melt remaining butter in the skillet and add garlic, cheese, heavy cream and spinach.

4. Cook for about 2 minutes and transfer the chicken in it.

5. Cook for about minutes on low heat and dish out to immediately serve.

6. Place chicken in a dish and set aside to cool for meal prepping. Divide it in 2 containers and cover them. Refrigerate for about 3 days and reheat in microwave before serving.

Nutrition Info: Calories: 288 ;Carbohydrates: 3.6g;Protein: 27g;Fat: 18.3g;Sugar: 0.3g;Sodium: 192mg

Niçoise-style Tuna Salad With Olives & White Beans

Servings: 4

Cooking Time: 20-30 Minutes

Ingredients:

- Green beans (.75 lb.)

- Solid white albacore tuna (12 oz. can)

- Great Northern beans (16 oz. can)

- Sliced black olives (2.25 oz.)

- Thinly sliced medium red onion (¼ of 1)

- Hard-cooked eggs (4 large)

- Dried oregano (1 tsp.)

- Olive oil (6 tbsp.)

- Black pepper and salt (as desired)

- Finely grated lemon zest (.5 tsp.)

- Water (.33 cup)

- Lemon juice (3 tbsp.)

Directions:

1. Drain the can of tuna, Great Northern beans, and black olives. Trim and snap the green beans into halves. Thinly slice the red onion. Cook and peel the eggs until hard-boiled.

2. Pour the water and salt into a skillet and add the beans. Place a top on the pot and switch the temperature setting to high. Wait for it to boil.

3. Once the beans are cooking, set a timer for five minutes. Immediately, drain and add the beans to a cookie sheet with a raised edge on paper towels to cool.

4. Combine the onion, olives, white beans, and drained tuna. Mix them with the zest, lemon juice, oil, and oregano.

5. Dump the mixture over the salad and gently toss.

6. Adjust the seasonings to your liking. Portion the tuna-bean salad with the green beans and eggs to serve.

Nutrition Info: Calories: 548;Protein: 36.3 grams;Fat: 30.3 grams

Whole-wheat Pasta With Roasted Red Pepper Sauce And Fresh Mozzarella

Servings: 4

Cooking Time: 40 Minutes

Ingredients:

- 3 large red bell peppers, seeds removed and cut in half

- 1 (10-ounce) container cherry tomatoes

- 2 teaspoons olive oil, plus 2 tablespoons

- 8 ounces whole-wheat penne or rotini

- 1 tablespoon plus 1 teaspoon apple cider vinegar

- 1 teaspoon chopped garlic

- 1½ teaspoons smoked paprika

- ¼ teaspoon kosher salt

- ½ cup packed fresh basil leaves, chopped

- 1 (8-ounce) container fresh whole-milk mozzarella balls (ciliegine), quartered

Directions:

1. Preheat the oven to 400°F and line a sheet pan with a silicone baking mat or parchment paper.

2. Place the peppers and tomatoes on the pan and toss with teaspoons of oil. Roast for 40 minutes.

3. While the peppers and tomatoes are roasting, cook the pasta according to the instructions on the box. Drain and place the pasta in a large mixing bowl.

4. When the peppers are cool enough to handle, peel the skin and discard. It's okay if you can't remove all the skin. Place the roasted peppers, vinegar, garlic, paprika, and salt and the remaining 2 tablespoons of oil in a blender and blend until smooth.

5. Add the pepper sauce, whole roasted tomatoes, basil, and mozzarella to the pasta and stir to combine.

6. Place a heaping 2 cups of pasta and sauce in each of 4 containers.

7. STORAGE: Store covered containers in the refrigerator for up to 5 days.

Nutrition Info:Per Serving: Total calories: 463; Total fat: 20g; Saturated fat: 7g; Sodium: 260mg; Carbohydrates: 54g; Fiber: 9g; Protein: 1

Greek Turkey Meatball Gyro With Tzatziki

Servings: 4

Cooking Time: 16 Minutes

Ingredients:

- Turkey Meatball:

- 1 lb. ground turkey

- 1/4 cup finely diced red onion

- 2 garlic cloves, minced

- 1 tsp oregano

- 1 cup chopped fresh spinach

- Salt, to taste

- Pepper, to taste

- 2 tbsp olive oil

- Tzatziki Sauce:

- 1/2 cup plain Greek yogurt

- 1/4 cup grated cucumber

- 2 tbsp lemon juice

- 1/2 tsp dry dill

- 1/2 tsp garlic powder

- Salt, to taste

- 1/2 cup thinly sliced red onion

- 1 cup diced tomato

- 1 cup diced cucumber

- 4 whole wheat flatbreads

Directions:

1. In a large bowl, add in ground turkey, diced red onion, oregano, fresh spinach minced garlic, salt, and pepper

2. Using your hands mix all the ingredients together until the meat forms a ball and sticks together

3. Then using your hands, form meat mixture into 1" balls, making about 12 meatballs

4. In a large skillet over medium high heat, add the olive oil and then add the meatballs, cook each side for 3-minutes until they are browned on all sides, remove from the pan and allow it to rest

5. Allow the dish to cool completely

6. Distribute in the container, store for 2-3 days

7. To Serve: Reheat in the microwave for 1-2 minutes or until heated through. In the

meantime, in a small bowl, combine the Greek yogurt, grated cucumber, lemon juice, dill, garlic powder, and salt to taste Assemble the gyros by taking the toasted flatbread, add 3 meatballs, sliced red onion, tomato, and cucumber. Top with Tzatziki sauce and serve!

Nutrition Info:Per Serving: Calories:429;Carbs: 3;Total Fat: 19g;Protein: 28g

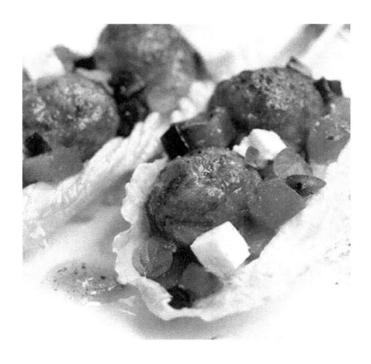

Grilled Mediterranean Chicken Kebabs

Servings: 10

Cooking Time: 10 Minutes

Ingredients:

- Chicken Kebabs:

- 3 chicken fillets, cut in 1-inch cubes

- 2 red bell peppers

- 2 green bell peppers

- 1 red onion

- Chicken Kebab Marinade:

- 2/3 cup extra virgin olive oil, divided

- Juice of 1 lemon, divided

- 6 clove of garlic, chopped, divided

- 4 tsp salt, divided

- 2 tsp freshly ground black pepper, divided

- 2 tsp paprika, divided

- 2 tsp thyme, divided

- 4 tsp oregano, divided

Directions:

1. In a bowl, mix 2 of all ingredients for the marinade- olive oils, lemon juice, garlic, salt, pepper, paprika, thyme and oregano in small bowl

2. Place the chicken in a ziplock bag and pour marinade over it, marinade in the fridge for about 30 minutes

3. In a separate ziplock bag, mix the other half of the marinade ingredients - olive oils, lemon juice, garlic, salt, pepper, paprika, thyme and

oregano - add the vegetables and marinade for at least minutes

4. If you are using wood skewers, soak the skewers in water for about 20-30 minutes

5. Once done, thread the chicken and peppers and onions on the skewers in a pattern about 6 pieces of chicken with peppers and onion in between

6. Over an outdoor grill or indoor grill pan over medium-high heat, spray the grates lightly with oil

7. Grill the chicken for about 5 minutes on each side, or until cooked through, then allow to cool completely

8. Distribute among the containers, store for 2-3 days

9. To Serve: Reheat in the microwave for 1-2 minutes or until heated through, or cover in foil

and reheat in the oven at 375 degrees F for 5 minutes

10. Recipe Notes: You can also bake the Mediterranean chicken skewers in the oven. Just preheat the oven to 425 F and place the chicken skewers on roasting racks that are over two foil-lined baking sheets. Bake for 15 minutes, turn over and bake for an additional 10 - 15 minutes on the other side, or until cooked through

Nutrition Info:Per Serving: Calories:228;Carbs: 5g;Total Fat: 17g;Protein: 14g

Kidney Beans Cilantro Salad

Servings: 6

Cooking Time: 30 Minutes

Ingredients:

- 1 15-ounce can kidney beans, rinsed and drained

- ½ English cucumber, chopped

- 1 medium heirloom tomato, chopped

- 1 bunch fresh cilantro, stems removed and chopped (about 1¼ cups)

- 1 red onion, chopped

- lime juice, 1 large lime

- 3 tablespoons Dijon mustard

- ½ teaspoon fresh garlic paste

- 1 teaspoon sumac

- salt

- pepper

Directions:

1. Place kidney beans, vegetables, and cilantro in a serving bowl.

2. Cover, refrigerate and allow it to chill.

3. Before serving, in a small bowl, make the vinaigrette by adding limejuice, oil, fresh garlic, pepper, mustard, and sumac.

4. Pour the vinaigrette over the salad and give it a gentle stir.

5. Add some salt and pepper.

6. Serve!

Nutrition Info:Per Serving: Calories: 269, Total Fat: 1.3 g, Saturated Fat: 0.2 g, Cholesterol: 0 mg,

Sodium: 112 mg, Total Carbohydrate: 49.3 g, Dietary Fiber: 12.g, Total Sugars: 3.9 g, Protein: 17.6 g, Vitamin D: 0 mcg, Calcium: 94 mg, Iron: 6 mg, Potassium: 1258 mg

Barley And Mushroom Soup

Servings: 6

Cooking Time: 30 Minutes

Ingredients:

- 2 tablespoons of olive oil

- 1 cup chopped carrots

- 6 cups vegetable broth, no salt added, and low sodium is best

- ¼ cup red wine

- 5 tablespoons parmesan cheese, grated

- ½ teaspoon thyme

- 1 cup chopped onion

- 5 cups chopped mushrooms

- 1 cup pearled barley, uncooked

- 2 tablespoons tomato paste

Directions:

1. Place a stockpot on your stove and turn the temperature of the range to medium heat.

2. Pour in the oil and let it warm up and start to simmer.

3. Combine the carrots and onion. Let them cook for 5 to 8 minutes while frequently stirring the ingredients together.

4. Add the mushroom and turn the heat up to medium-high. Stir and cook for a few minutes.

5. Pour in the broth and stir the ingredients for a few seconds.

6. Add in the wine, barley, thyme, and tomato paste. Stir everything together and then set the cover on the pot.

7. When the soup starts to boil, stir and reduce the heat to medium-low.

8. Cover the soup again and set your timer for 15 minutes, but don't leave it alone. You will want to stir a few times, so all ingredients become well incorporated.

9. Once the dish becomes fragrant and the barley is completely cooked, turn off the heat and serve in bowls. Sprinkle the cheese on top for added taste and enjoy!

Nutrition Info: calories: 236, fats: 7 grams, carbohydrates: 35 grams, protein: 8 grams.

Pan-seared Scallops With Pepper & Onions In Anchovy Oil

Servings: 4

Cooking Time: 45 Minutes

Ingredients:

- Olive oil (.33 cup)

- Anchovy fillets (2 oz. can)

- Jumbo sea scallops (1 lb.)

- Orange & red bell pepper (1 large of each)

- Red onion (1)

- Garlic (2 cloves)

- Lime zest (1 tsp.)

- Lemon zest (1.5 tsp.)

- Kosher salt & pepper (1 pinch of each)

- Garnish: Fresh parsley (8 sprigs)

Directions:

1. Coarsely chop the peppers and onions. Mince the garlic and anchovy fillet. Zest/mince the lime and lemon.

2. Heat the oil and anchovies in a large skillet using a med-high temperature setting.

3. After the anchovies are sizzling, toss in the scallops, and simmer them for about two minutes - without stirring.

4. Toss the bell peppers, garlic, red onion, lime zest, lemon zest, salt, and pepper into a mixing container. Sprinkle the mixture over the scallops. Cook until they have browned (2 min..)

5. Flip the scallops, stir, and continue cooking until the scallops have browned thoroughly (4-min..)

6. Top it off using sprigs of parsley before serving.

Nutrition   Info: Calories: 368;Protein: 24.2 grams;Fat: 23.9 grams

Chicken Sausage, Artichoke, Kale, And White Bean Gratin

Servings: 8

Cooking Time: 45 Minutes

Ingredients:

- 2 teaspoons olive oil, plus 2 tablespoons

- 1 small yellow onion, chopped (about 2 cups)

- 1 (12-ounce) package fully cooked chicken-apple sausage, sliced

- 1 bunch kale, stemmed and chopped (6 to 7 cups)

- ½ cup dry white wine, such as sauvignon blanc

- 4 ounces soft goat cheese

- 2 (15.5-ounce) cans cannellini or great northern beans, drained and rinsed

- 1 (14-ounce) can quartered artichoke hearts

- 1 (14.5-ounce) can no-salt-added diced tomatoes

- 1 teaspoon herbes de Provence

- ¼ teaspoon kosher salt

- 1 cup panko bread crumbs

- 1 teaspoon garlic powder

Directions:

1. Preheat the oven to 350°F. Lightly oil a -by-9-inch glass or ceramic baking dish.

2. Heat teaspoons of oil in a 12-inch skillet over medium-high heat. When the oil is shimmering, add the onion and cook for 2 minutes. Add the sausage and brown for 3 minutes. Add the kale and cook until wilted, about 3 more minutes. Add the wine and cook for 1 additional minute.

3. Add the goat cheese and stir until it is melted and the mixture looks creamy.

4. Add the beans, artichokes, tomatoes, herbes de Provence, and salt, and stir to combine. Transfer the contents of the pan to the baking dish.

5. Mix the bread crumbs, the garlic powder, and the remaining 2 tablespoons of oil in a small bowl. Spread the bread crumbs evenly across the top of the casserole.

6. Cover the dish with foil and bake for 30 minutes. Remove the foil and bake for 15 more minutes, until the bread crumbs are lightly browned. Cool.

7. Place about 1½ cups of casserole in each of 8 containers.

8. STORAGE: Store covered containers in the refrigerator for up to 5 days. Gratin can be frozen for up to 3 months.

Nutrition Info:Per Serving: Total calories: 367; Total fat: 14g; Saturated fat: 5g; Sodium: 624mg; Carbohydrates: 40g; Fiber: 10g; Protein: 1

Spinach Salad With Blood Orange Vinaigrette

Servings: 6

Cooking Time: 10 Minutes

Ingredients:

- ½ cup fresh blood orange juice

- 1/3 cup extra-virgin olive oil

- 2 tablespoons sherry reserve vinegar

- 1 tablespoon fresh grated ginger

- 1 teaspoon garlic powder

- 1 teaspoon ground sumac

- salt

- pepper

- 1/3 cup dried apricots, chopped

- 2 tablespoons sherry reserve vinegar

- 2 loaves pita bread

- 2/3 cup vegetable oil

- 1/3 cup raw unsalted almonds

- 1/3 cup raw sliced almonds

- ½ teaspoon sumac

- ½ teaspoon paprika

- salt

- 4 cups baby spinach

- 3 cups frisee lettuce, chopped

- 2 shallots, thinly sliced

- 1-2 blood oranges, peeled and sliced crosswise

Directions:

1. In a small bowl, soak the dried apricots in the sherry-reserved vinegar for about 5 minutes.

2. Drain apricots and set aside.

3. Toast pita bread until crispy and break into pieces.

4. Heat vegetable oil in a frying pan over medium-high heat.

5. Add broken pitas and almonds and fry them for a while.

6. Add sliced up almonds, sumac, and paprika, and toss everything well.

7. Remove from heat once the almonds show a golden brown color.

8. Place on paper towels and allow to drain.

9. In a mixing bowl, add baby spinach, shallots, apricots, frisee lettuce.

10. Prepare the vinaigrette by taking a bowl and whisking in all blood orange vinaigrette Ingredients: listed above.

11. Before serving, dress the salad with the prepared orange vinaigrette and toss well.

12. Add fried pita chips and almonds and toss again.

13. Serve into individual bowls with a garnish of two blood orange slices.

14. Enjoy!

Nutrition Info:Per Serving: Calories: 462, Total Fat: 41.2 g, Saturated Fat: 6.9 g, Cholesterol: 0 mg, Sodium: 110 mg, Total Carbohydrate: 22.6 g, Dietary Fiber: 6.8 g, Total Sugars: 6.8 g, Protein: 6.1 g, Vitamin D: 0 mcg, Calcium: 163 mg, Iron: 3 mg, Potassium: 702 mg

Lasagna Tortellini Soup

Servings: 6

Cooking Time: 6 Hours

Ingredients:

- 1 lb extra lean ground beef

- 1 package (16 oz) frozen cheese filled tortellini

- 3 cups beef broth

- 1/2 cup yellow onion, chopped

- 2 cloves garlic, minced

- 1 can (28 oz) crushed tomatoes

- 1 can (14.5 oz) petite diced tomatoes

- 1 can (6 oz) tomato paste

- 1 can (10.75 oz) tomato condensed soup

- 1 tsp white sugar

- 1 ½ tsp dried basil

- 1 tsp Italian seasoning

- 1/2 tbsp salt, to taste

- 1/4 tsp pepper

- Optional:

- 4 tbsp fresh parsley

- 1/2 tsp fennel seeds

- Toppings:

- Freshly grated Parmesan cheese

- Large spoonful of ricotta cheese

Directions:

1. In a large skillet over medium heat, brown the ground beef until cooked through

2. Add the onion and garlic in the last few minutes of the cooking

3. While the beef is cooking, pour in the crushed tomatoes, petite diced tomatoes, tomato paste, and tomato condensed soup in the slow cooker. - Don't drain the cans!

4. Add in the sugar, the dried basil, fennel, Italian seasoning, salt, and pepper, adjust to taste

5. Stir in the cooked ground beef with onions and garlic

6. Add in the beef broth – or dissolved beef bouillon cubes into boiling water

7. Cook on high for 3-4 hours or low for 5-hours.

8. 15-20 minutes before you are ready to serve the soup, add in the frozen tortellini

9. Set the slow cooker to high and allow the tortellini to heat through

10. Allow to cool, then distribute the soup into the container and store in the fridge for up to 3 days

11. To Serve: Reheat in the microwave or on the stove top, top with freshly grated Parmesan cheese, a large spoonful of ricotta cheese, extra seasonings and freshly chopped parsley.

Nutrition Info:Per Serving: Calories:499;Total Fat: 17g;Total Carbs: 53g;Fiber: 8g;Protein: 34g

Greek Quinoa Bowls

Servings: 2

Cooking Time: 12 Minutes

Ingredients:

- 1 cup quinoa

- 1 ½ cups water

- 1 cup chopped green bell pepper

- 1 cup chopped red bell pepper

- 1/3 cup crumbled feta cheese

- 1/4 cup extra virgin olive oil

- 2-3 tbsp apple cider vinegar

- Salt, to taste

- Pepper, to taste

- 1-2 tbsp fresh parsley

- To Serve:

- Hummus

- Pita wedges

- Olives

- Fresh tomatoes

- Sliced or chopped avocado

- Lemon wedges

Directions:

1. Rinse and drain the quinoa using a mesh strainer or sieve. Place a medium saucepan to medium heat and lightly toast the quinoa to remove any excess water. Stir as it toasts for just a few minutes, to add a nuttiness and fluff to the quinoa

2. Then add the water, set burner to high, and bring to a boil.

3. Once boiling, reduce heat to low and simmer, covered with the lid slightly ajar, for 12-1minutes or until quinoa is fluffy and the liquid have been absorbed

4. In the meantime, mix whisk together olive oil, apple cider vinegar, salt, and pepper to make the dressing, store in the fridge until ready to serve

5. Add in the red bell peppers, green bell peppers, and parsley

6. Give the quinoa a little fluff with a fork, remove from the pot

7. Allow to cool completely

8. Distribute among the containers, store for 2-3 days

9. To Serve: Reheat in the microwave for 1-2 minutes or until heated through.

10. Pour the dressing over the quinoa bowl, toss add the feta cheese. Season with additional salt and pepper to taste, if desired. Enjoy!

Nutrition Info:Per Serving: Calories:645;Carbs: 61g;Total Fat: 37g;Protein: 16g

Salmon Stew

Servings: 2

Cooking Time: 20 Minutes

Ingredients:

- 1 pound salmon fillet, sliced

- 1 onion, chopped

- Salt, to taste

- 1 tablespoon butter, melted

- 1 cup fish broth

- ½ teaspoon red chili powder

Directions:

1. Season the salmon fillets with salt and red chili powder.

2. Put butter and onions in a skillet and sauté for about 3 minutes.

3. Add seasoned salmon and cook for about 2 minutes on each side.

4. Add fish broth and secure the lid.

5. Cook for about 7 minutes on medium heat and open the lid.

6. Dish out and serve immediately.

7. Transfer the stew in a bowl and keep aside to cool for meal prepping. Divide the mixture into 2 containers. Cover the containers and refrigerate for about 2 days. Reheat in the microwave before serving.

Nutrition Info: Calories: 272 ;Carbohydrates: 4.4g;Protein: 32.1g;Fat: 14.2g   ;Sugar: 1.9g;Sodium: 275mg

Balsamic Chicken And Veggie Skewers

Servings: 4

Cooking Time: 25 Minutes

Ingredients:

- 1 pound boneless, skinless chicken breasts, cut into 1-inch cubes

- ⅓ cup balsamic vinegar

- 4 tablespoons olive oil, divided

- 4 teaspoons dried Italian herbs, divided

- 2 teaspoons garlic powder, divided

- 2 teaspoons onion powder, divided

- 8 ounces whole button or cremini mushrooms, stems removed

- 1 large red bell pepper, cut into 1-inch squares

- 1 small red onion, quartered and layers pulled apart

- 1 large zucchini, sliced into ½-inch rounds

- ¾ teaspoon kosher salt

- 8 (11¾-inch) wooden or metal skewers, soaked in water for at least 1 hour if wooden

Directions:

1. Preheat the oven to 450°F. Line a sheet pan with aluminum foil.

2. Place the chicken in a gallon-size resealable bag along with the balsamic vinegar, tablespoons of oil, 2 teaspoons of Italian herbs, 1 teaspoon of garlic powder, and 1 teaspoon of onion powder. Seal the bag and make sure all the pieces of chicken are coated with marinade.

3. In a second resealable bag, place the mushrooms, bell pepper, onion, and zucchini and the remaining 2 tablespoons of oil, 2

teaspoons of Italian herbs, 1 teaspoon of garlic powder, and 1 teaspoon of onion powder. Seal the bag and shake to make sure the veggies are coated.

4. Refrigerate both bags and marinate for at least 2 hours.

5. Thread the chicken and veggies on 8 skewers, alternating both chicken and veggies on each skewer. Place 6 skewers vertically in the center of the pan, 1 horizontally at the top, and 1 at the bottom. Sprinkle half the salt over the skewers, then flip over and sprinkle the skewers with the remaining salt.

6. Bake for 15 minutes, carefully flip the skewers, then bake for another 10 minutes. Cool.

7. If you have containers long enough to fit the skewers, place 2 skewers directly in each of 4 containers. If not, break the skewers in half or slide the meat and veggies off the skewers.

8. STORAGE: Store covered containers in the refrigerator for up to 5 days.

Nutrition Info:Per Serving: Total calories: 224; Total fat: 10g; Saturated fat: 2g; Sodium: 631mg; Carbohydrates: 11g; Fiber: 3g; Protein: 27g

Pesto Chicken And Tomato Zoodles

Servings: 4

Cooking Time: 15 Minutes

Ingredients:

- 3 Zucchini, inspiralized

- 2 boneless skinless chicken breasts

- 1 1/2 cup cherry tomatoes

- 2 tsp olive oil

- 1/2 tsp salt

- Store brought Pesto or Homemade Basil Pesto

- Salt, to taste

- Pepper, to taste

Directions:

1. Preheat grill to medium high heat

2. Season both sides of the chicken with salt and pepper

3. Place cherry tomatoes in a small bowl, add the olive oil and 1/2 tsp salt, and toss the tomatoes

4. In the meantime, inspiralize the zucchini, set aside

5. Pour the pesto over the zucchini noodles, using salad toss or tongs, mix the pesto in with the zoodles until it is completely combined

6. Place the chicken on the grill and grill each side for 5-7 minutes, or until cooked through

7. Place cherry tomatoes in a grill basket and grill for 5 minutes, until tomatoes burst

8. Remove the tomatoes and chicken from the grill, slice the chicken and place both sliced chicken and tomatoes into the pesto zoodles bowl

9. allow the dish to cool completely

10. Distribute among the containers, store for 2-3 days

11. To Serve: Reheat in the microwave for 1-2 minutes or until heated through. Enjoy

Nutrition Info:Per Serving: Calories:396;Carbs: 8g;Total Fat: 30g;Protein: 18g

Conclusion

We've come to the end of this wonderful journey, did you delight in these fantastic recipes?

Is your family happy?

Work out and cook these delicacies every day, adopting a Mediterranean eating style is good for your health and spirit.

Thank you and I embrace you.